Mindful Mastery:

A guide to

Mental

Health

Strategies

Mitchell Coren

Foreword: Castor Mann

Credits

Amazon KDP.com

Pexels.com

Canva.com

Dedication

To the brave souls who have faced mental storms and those still finding their way through, this book is dedicated to your strength and resilience.

You are not alone.

Foreword

*In the realm of self-discovery and mental well-being,
"Mindful Mastery: Mental Health Strategies" emerges as a
beacon of enlightenment. Mitchell Coren, with profound
insight and empathetic prose, takes us on a transformative
expedition through the corridors of the mind.*

*As you turn these pages, be prepared to embark on a holistic
journey—one that weaves together the threads of
psychology, mindfulness, and the human experience.

Writer's thoughtful exploration provides not only a roadmap
for navigating mental health challenges but also a compelling
narrative that resonates on a profound level.*

*In "Mindful Mastery," you'll discover more than a guide;
you'll find a companion—a trusted ally in the pursuit of a
balanced and fulfilling life. I am honored to introduce you to
a work that transcends the boundaries of self-help, offering a
genuine and compassionate approach to the pursuit of
mental well-being.*

[Dr. Castor Mann]

TABLE OF CONTENTS

Introduction

In the hustle and bustle of our modern lives, the significance of mental health often takes a backseat amidst the daily chaos.

Welcome to "Mindful Mastery: A Guide to Mental Health Strategies," where we embark on a journey to unravel the profound importance of nurturing our mental well-being.

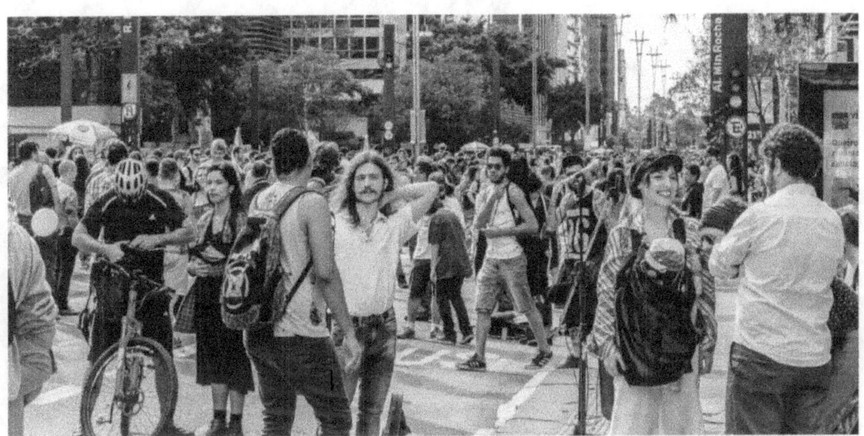

The Importance of Mental Health

Our mental health is the silent conductor orchestrating the symphony of our lives. Just as physical health is paramount, so too is the well-being of our minds. In this introduction, we delve into the fundamental reasons why mental health is not merely an aspect of our lives but the very essence that colors our experiences. From the ebbs and flows of our emotions to the clarity of our thoughts, every facet of our existence is intricately woven into the tapestry of mental health.

Understanding Common Mental Health Challenges

Acknowledging the importance of mental health requires an honest exploration of the challenges that many encounter on this intricate journey. Anxiety, depression, and various other mental health challenges are not uncommon companions in our lives. In this section, we unravel the threads of these common challenges, offering insights and understanding to foster empathy and awareness.

As we embark on this exploration, keep in mind that this guide is not just about understanding; it is a roadmap to mindful mastery—an empowering voyage toward a resilient and flourishing mental landscape. Join us as we navigate the intricacies of the mind, providing tools and strategies to cultivate a profound sense of well-being.

Chapter 1: Building a Foundation for Mental Wellness

Mind-Body Connection

The mind and body dance in an intricate partnership, each influencing the other in a profound symbiosis. In this chapter, we explore the fascinating realm of the mind-body connection, unraveling the ways in which our thoughts and emotions impact our physical well-being, and vice versa. From the subtle interplay of neurotransmitters to the tangible effects of stress on the body, we delve into the science and art of fostering a harmonious mind-body relationship.

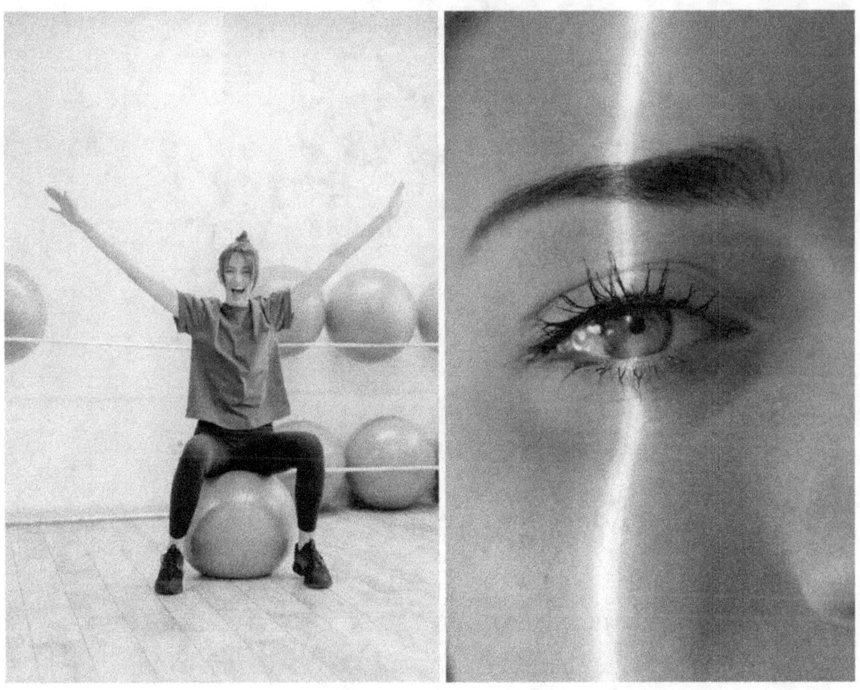

Establishing Healthy Habits

At the core of mental wellness lies the foundation of daily habits. This section is a practical guide to cultivating habits that nurture mental health. From the rhythm of sleep to the fuel we provide our bodies, every choice contributes to the resilience of our minds. Through actionable insights, we empower you to establish habits that not only fortify mental well-being but also create a sustainable framework for a fulfilling life.

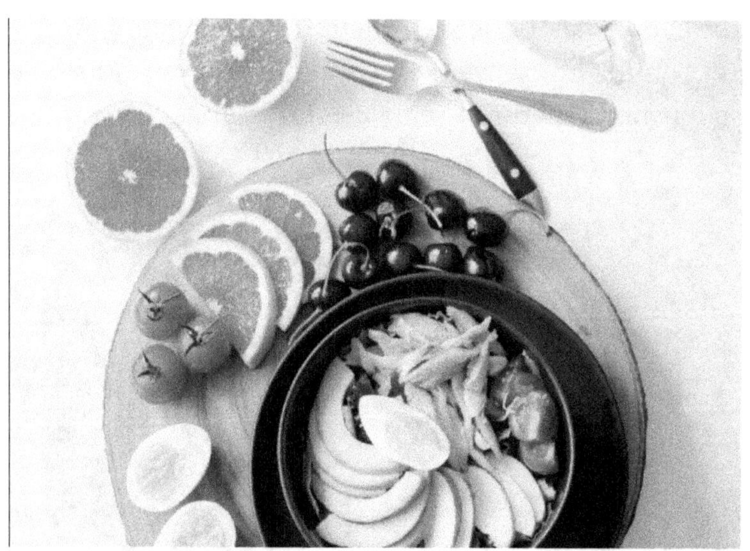

Stress Management Techniques

Stress, an inevitable companion on life's journey, requires a skillful response for mental equilibrium. Here, we introduce an arsenal of stress management techniques, ranging from mindfulness practices to proven relaxation methods. Uncover the power of breath in anchoring the mind, learn to navigate the turbulent waters of stress with resilience, and discover personalized strategies that resonate with your unique journey. As we navigate the complexities of stress, remember that this chapter serves as a toolbox, providing you with the instruments to craft a serene and resilient mental landscape.

In "Mindful Mastery," Chapter 1 is not merely an introduction; it's a blueprint for crafting a foundation that sustains and uplifts your mental well-being. Join us as we lay the groundwork for a transformative journey towards a more resilient, balanced, and mindful life.

Chapter 2: Nurturing Emotional Well-Being

Embracing Emotions

Our emotions, the vibrant colors of the human experience, deserve not only acknowledgment but also a compassionate embrace. In this chapter, we navigate the intricate tapestry of emotions, exploring their nuances and uncovering the transformative power of embracing them. By fostering a healthy relationship with our emotions, we pave the way for greater emotional resilience and well-being.

Cultivating Resilience

Life's journey is a series of ebbs and flows, and resilience is the compass that guides us through both triumphs and tribulations. Here, we delve into the art of cultivating resilience—a key pillar of emotional well-being. Through stories of triumph over adversity and practical strategies, this section empowers you to navigate life's challenges with a spirit that not only withstands but also flourishes.

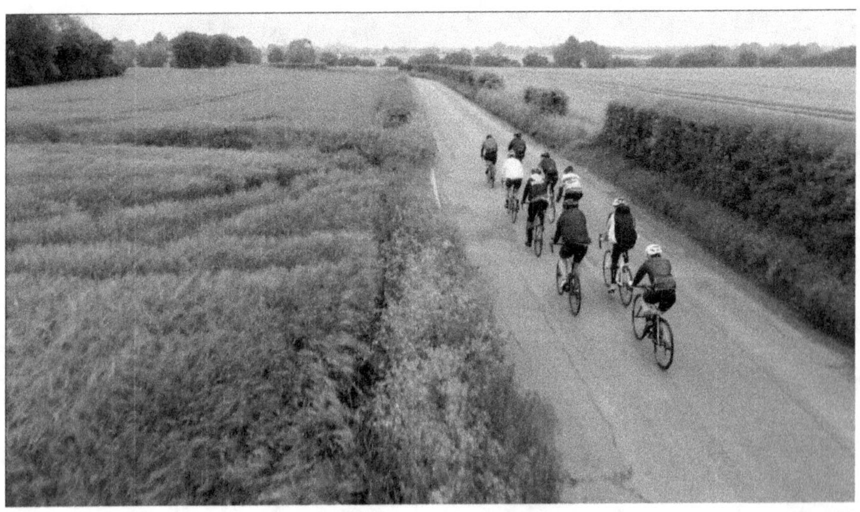

Positive Psychology Approaches

Positivity is not just a fleeting sentiment but a powerful force that shapes our outlook on life. Positive psychology, the science of happiness and flourishing, takes center stage in this section. Discover evidence-based approaches to enhance your well-being, foster a positive mindset, and cultivate a life filled with meaning and purpose. As we explore these approaches, remember that nurturing emotional well-being is not about eliminating challenges but about transforming our relationship with them.

In "Mindful Mastery," Chapter 2 is a voyage into the heart of emotional well-being. Join us as we navigate the seas of emotions, strengthen the sails of resilience, and set a course toward a more positive and fulfilling life.

Chapter 3: Cognitive Strategies for Mental Clarity

Cognitive Behavioral Techniques

The mind, a labyrinth of thoughts and beliefs, plays a pivotal role in shaping our mental landscape. This chapter introduces the transformative world of cognitive behavioral techniques (CBT), providing a roadmap to navigate and reframe thought patterns. Uncover the power of identifying and challenging negative thoughts, cultivating a more positive cognitive framework that enhances mental clarity and well-being.

Mindfulness and Meditation

At the heart of mental clarity lies the practice of mindfulness and meditation. Dive deep into the art of being present, cultivating awareness of thoughts and sensations. Explore various meditation techniques that not only calm the mind but also promote a heightened sense of clarity and focus. Through mindfulness, discover the profound impact of living in the present moment on your overall mental well-being.

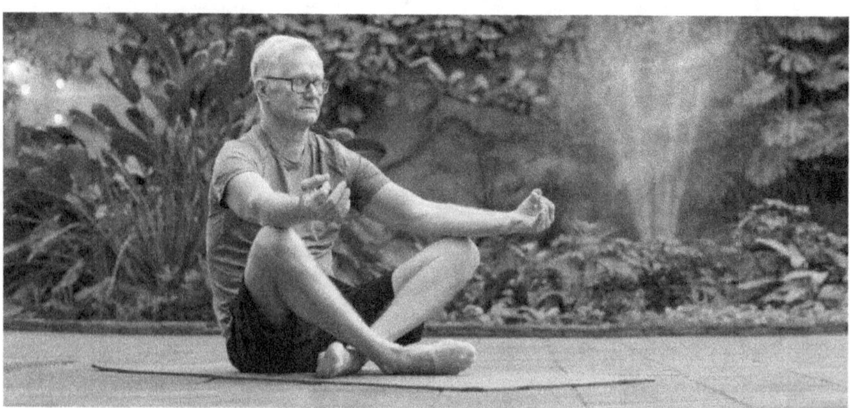

Enhancing Cognitive Flexibility

In a world of constant change, cognitive flexibility is a valuable asset. This section explores strategies to enhance cognitive flexibility—a dynamic mindset that adapts to new information and challenges. By embracing uncertainty and fostering a mindset open to different perspectives, you empower yourself to navigate the complexities of life with resilience and mental agility.

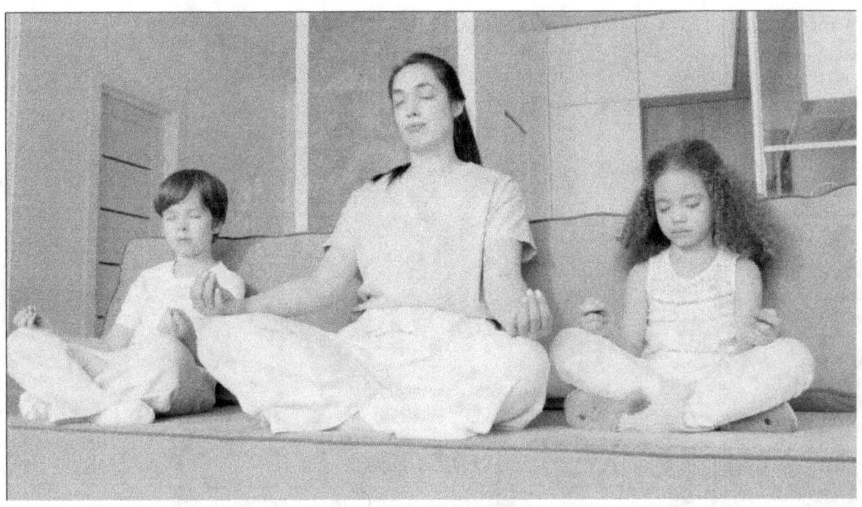

As we journey through "Mindful Mastery," Chapter 3 illuminates the path to mental clarity. From reshaping thought patterns to embracing the power of mindfulness, these cognitive strategies serve as a compass, guiding you toward a mind that is not only clear but also adaptable to the ever-evolving landscape of your experiences. Join us as we unravel the layers of the mind and cultivate a cognitive framework that fosters lasting mental well-being.

Chapter 4: Social Connections and Mental Health

Building Supportive Relationships

Human connection is the fabric that weaves together the tapestry of our lives. In this chapter, we delve into the profound impact of relationships on mental health. Explore the art of building supportive connections, nurturing friendships, and cultivating meaningful bonds that serve as pillars of strength during life's challenges. Discover the reciprocal nature of positive relationships and their transformative influence on your mental well-being.

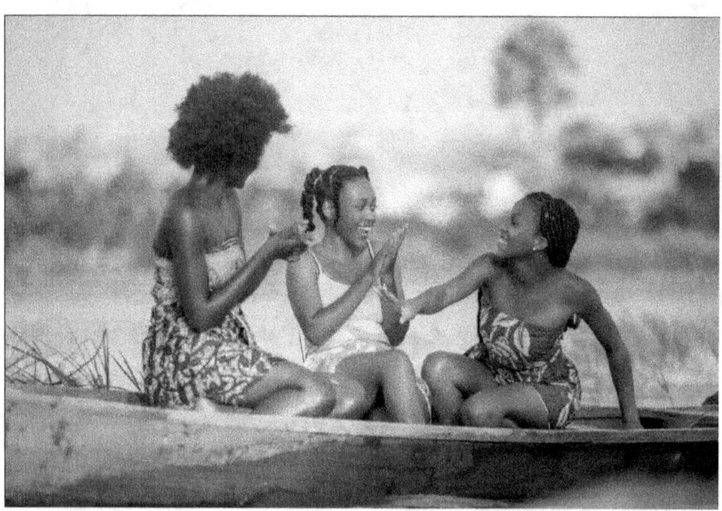

Communication Skills

Effective communication is the bridge that connects hearts and minds. This section focuses on honing communication skills to strengthen your interpersonal relationships. Learn to express yourself authentically, listen empathetically, and navigate conflicts with grace. These skills not only enhance the quality of your connections but also contribute to a more harmonious and emotionally fulfilling life.

Overcoming Social Isolation

In a digitally connected yet paradoxically isolating world, addressing social isolation is paramount. Explore strategies to overcome feelings of loneliness and foster a sense of belonging. Whether through community engagement, shared interests, or volunteering, discover avenues to connect with others and create a supportive social network that bolsters your mental health.

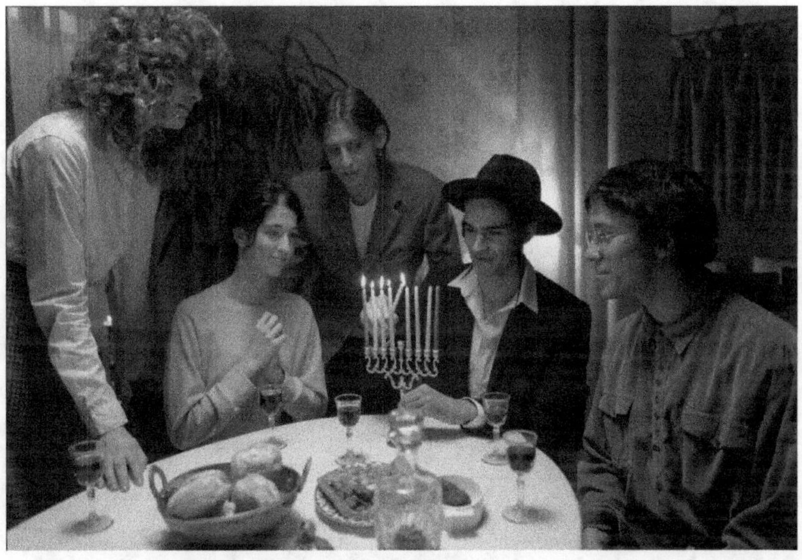

Chapter 4 of "Mindful Mastery" is a testament to the transformative power of social connections. Join us as we explore the profound impact of relationships, sharpen communication skills, and navigate the delicate dance of human connection. Through building a supportive social framework, you not only enrich your life but also cultivate a resilient mental landscape that thrives on the strength of meaningful connections.

Chapter 5: Lifestyle Factors Impacting Mental Health

Sleep Hygiene

Sleep, a cornerstone of well-being, plays a pivotal role in mental health. This chapter unravels the intricacies of sleep hygiene, offering insights into creating a sleep-friendly environment, establishing bedtime routines, and understanding the profound impact of quality sleep on mental clarity and emotional resilience. Explore practical strategies to enhance your sleep patterns and nurture a restorative night's sleep.

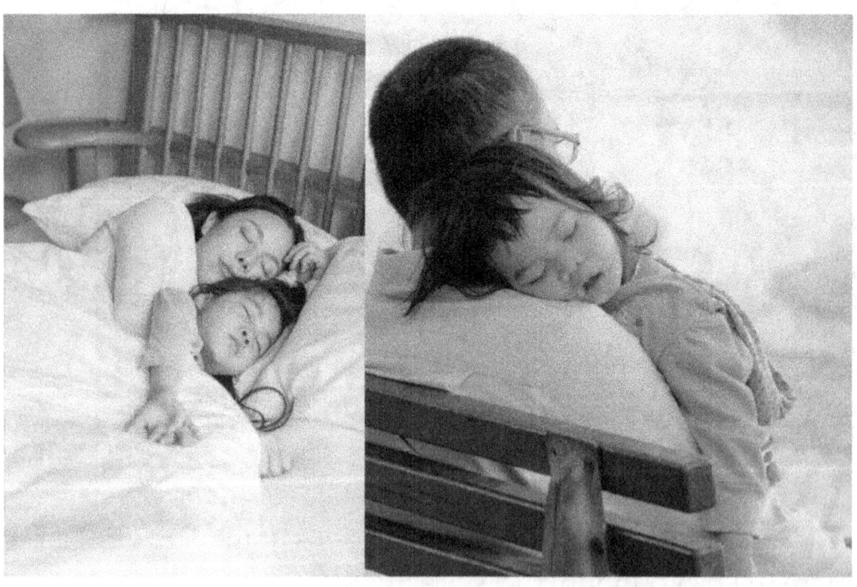

Nutrition for Brain Health

The fuel we provide our bodies directly influences the functioning of our minds. Delve into the connection between nutrition and mental health, exploring foods that support brain function and emotional well-being. From the importance of balanced meals to the role of specific nutrients, discover dietary practices that contribute to a healthy mind and body.

Physical Exercise and Mental Well-Being

Exercise is not just a means of physical fitness but a powerful tool for mental well-being. This section explores the synergistic relationship between physical activity and mental health. Uncover the mood-boosting benefits of exercise, explore different forms of physical activity, and learn how movement becomes a catalyst for reducing stress, enhancing cognitive function, and fostering overall mental resilience.

Chapter 5 of "Mindful Mastery" is a holistic exploration of lifestyle factors that impact mental health. Join us as we navigate the realms of sleep, nutrition, and exercise, recognizing that the choices we make in our daily lives profoundly influence our mental well-being. By embracing a lifestyle that prioritizes these factors, you lay the groundwork for a resilient and flourishing mental landscape.

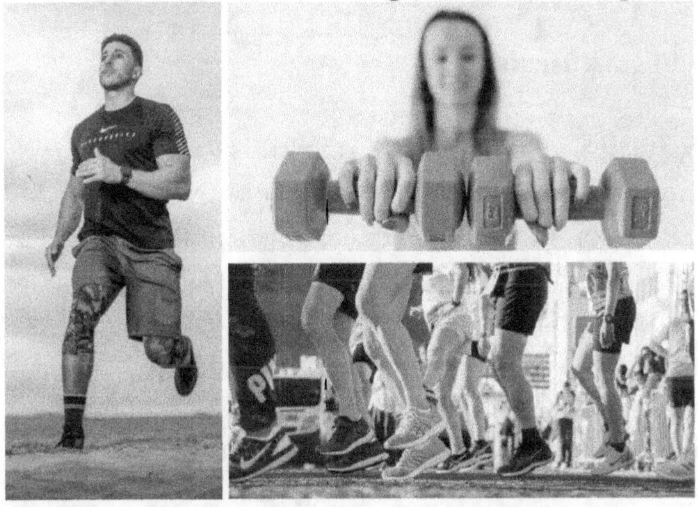

Chapter 6: Coping with Specific Challenges

Anxiety Management

Anxiety, a common companion on life's journey, requires a nuanced approach for effective management.

In this chapter, we delve into practical strategies to navigate anxiety. Explore mindfulness techniques, cognitive-behavioral tools, and relaxation exercises that empower you to understand, cope with, and ultimately transcend the challenges posed by anxiety. By fostering a proactive relationship with anxiety, you can transform it into a catalyst for personal growth and resilience.

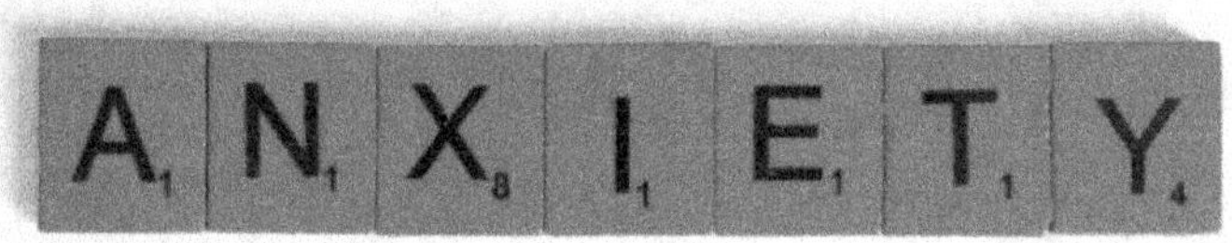

Depression Coping Strategies

Depression, often shrouded in silence, demands compassionate understanding and targeted coping strategies. This section guides you through practical approaches to cope with depression. From building a robust support system to incorporating mood-enhancing activities, discover techniques that empower you to navigate the complexities of depression. As we explore these strategies, remember that seeking help and implementing coping mechanisms are courageous steps toward healing.

Dealing with Trauma

Trauma, a profound impact on mental well-being, requires delicate navigation. This part of the chapter provides insights into understanding and addressing trauma. Explore therapeutic interventions, self-care practices, and resilience-building strategies to heal from the effects of trauma. By acknowledging and working through these experiences, you pave the way for a more resilient and empowered sense of self.

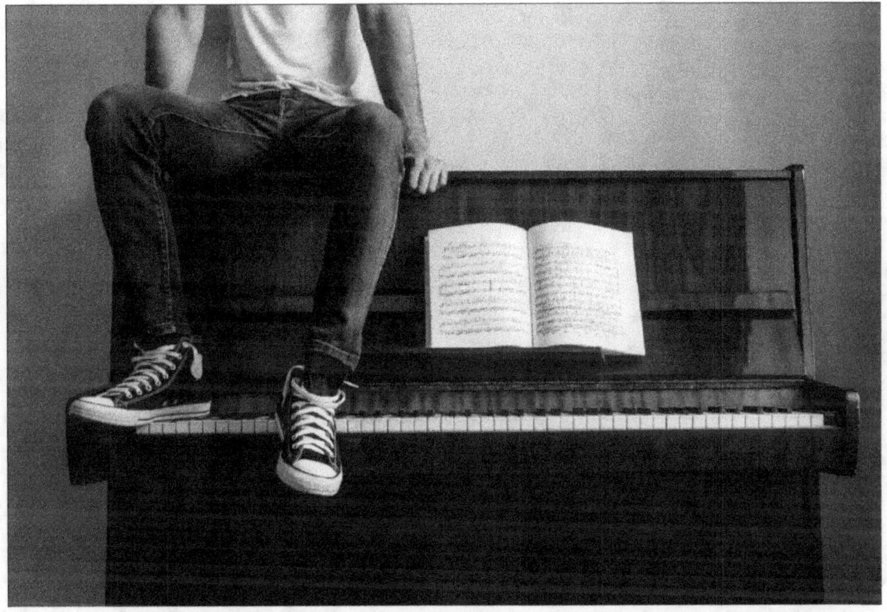

Chapter 6 of "Mindful Mastery" is a compassionate guide through the specific challenges that many encounter on their mental health journey. Join us as we explore practical coping strategies for anxiety, depression, and trauma, recognizing that each challenge is an opportunity for growth and healing.

Through understanding, empathy, and actionable tools, you can cultivate a resilient mindset that transcends adversities.

Chapter 7: Seeking Professional Help

In this crucial chapter, the focus is on acknowledging the significance of professional support in managing mental health.

The Importance of Therapy

Cognitive-Behavioral Therapy (CBT) focuses on thoughts and behaviors, while Psychodynamic Therapy delves into unconscious patterns. Mindfulness-Based Therapies enhance present moment awareness, and Humanistic Therapies emphasize personal growth and self-actualization.

Additionally, there's Dialectical Behavior Therapy (DBT) for emotional regulation and Family Systems Therapy for addressing relational dynamics.

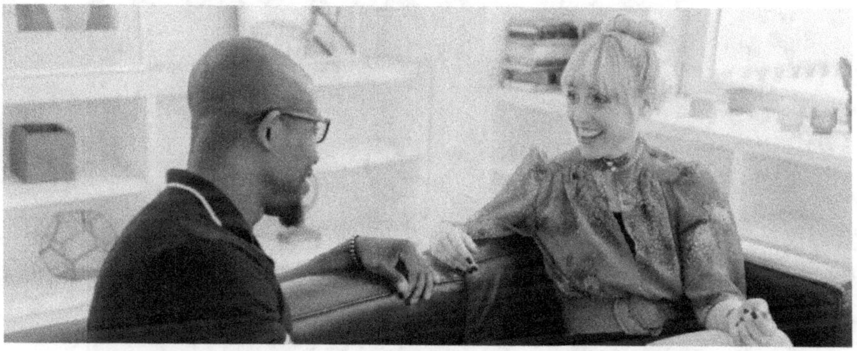

Medication and Mental Health

Medication can be a valuable tool in managing mental health, helping alleviate symptoms for many individuals. However, it's crucial to recognize that it's just one aspect of a comprehensive approach. Therapy, lifestyle changes, and support networks are equally important. Medication

addresses symptoms, while other strategies contribute to
long-term well-being and coping skills, creating a holistic
approach to mental health care.

Common psychiatric medications include antidepressants
(e.g., SSRIs, SNRIs), which can alleviate mood disorders, and
anxiolytics (e.g., benzodiazepines) for anxiety. Antipsychotics
(e.g., typical and atypical) treat psychosis. Mood stabilizers
(e.g., lithium) help with bipolar disorder, and stimulants (e.g.,
for ADHD) enhance focus. Potential benefits include
symptom relief, improved functioning, and enhanced quality
of life. However, side effects vary and may include weight
gain, drowsiness, or sexual dysfunction. Balancing benefits
and side effects is crucial, requiring close monitoring by
healthcare professionals.

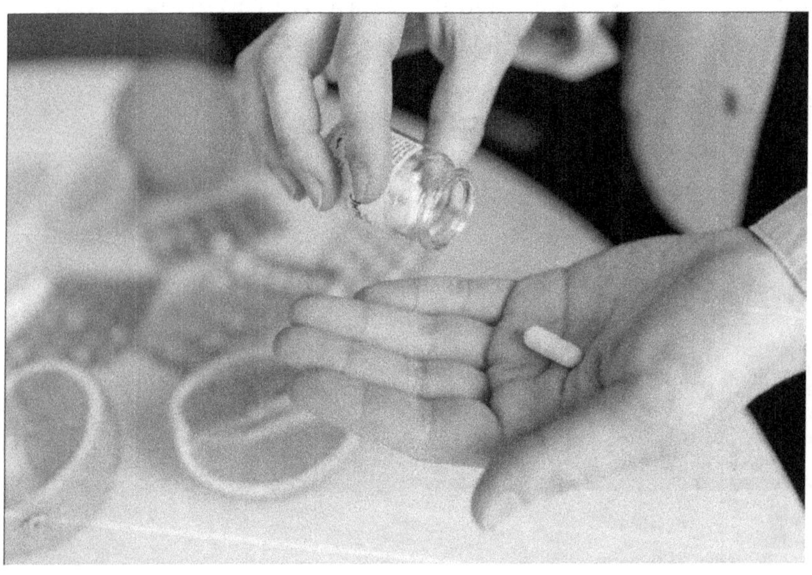

Finding the Right Mental Health Professional

Therapy provides a supportive environment to explore and
address mental health challenges, offering coping
mechanisms, emotional regulation, and tools for self-

discovery. It promotes better understanding of oneself and facilitates positive behavioral changes, contributing to overall mental well-being.

Therapeutic approaches vary, each tailored to specific needs.

Choosing the right therapist involves considering personal needs and preferences. Research their expertise, therapeutic approach, and experience with your concerns. Consider compatibility in terms of communication style and personality. Seek recommendations, read reviews, and schedule an initial consultation to gauge the connection. Trust your instincts; a strong therapeutic alliance is essential. Additionally, ensure the therapist's credentials align with your expectations and verify their licensing. Regularly assess progress and be open to reevaluating if the therapeutic relationship isn't meeting your needs.

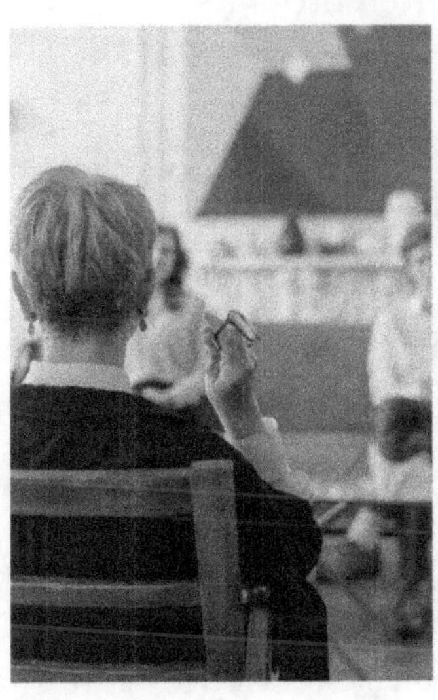
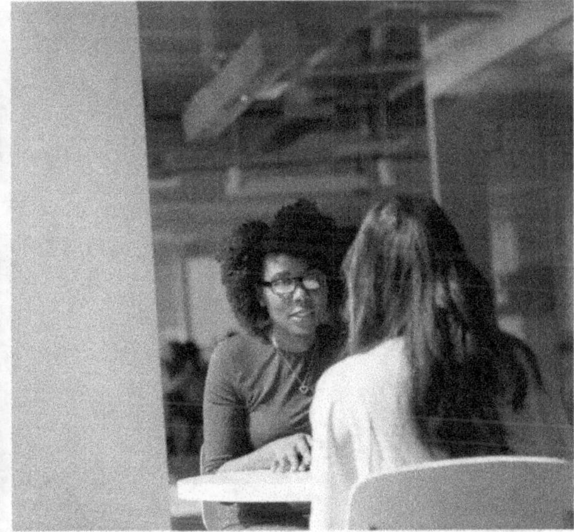

Practical tips on researching professionals, considering specialties and understanding therapeutic approaches

Online Directories: Use reputable online directories to find professionals in your area. Websites like Psychology Today or professional licensing boards provide details about therapists.

Specialties: Identify therapists with expertise in your specific concerns. Look for those with experience in areas such as anxiety, depression, or relationship issues.

Credentials: Verify their credentials and licensing. Ensure they have the appropriate qualifications to practice therapy in your location.

Reviews and Recommendations: Read client reviews and seek recommendations from friends, family, or healthcare providers. Personal referrals often provide valuable insights.

Initial Consultation: Schedule an initial consultation. This meeting allows you to assess the therapist's approach, ask questions, and determine if there's a comfortable rapport.

Therapeutic Approach: Research various therapeutic approaches (CBT, psychodynamic, etc.) and consider which aligns with your preferences. Discuss this with potential therapists to ensure a good fit.

Experience: Inquire about the therapist's experience with your specific issues. Experience can contribute to a deeper understanding and more effective treatment.

Payment and Insurance: Clarify payment details and check if they accept your insurance. Understand the financial aspect to ensure it aligns with your budget.

Flexibility: Consider the therapist's availability and scheduling options. Find someone whose availability matches your needs.

Gut Feeling: Trust your instincts during the research process. If something feels off or doesn't align with your preferences, it's okay to explore other options.

Seeking professional support is strength, not a weakness. Acknowledging the need for help and taking steps toward mental health is a courageous and proactive decision. Therapists are trained to provide guidance, support, and tools for navigating challenges. Just as one would consult a professional for physical health, recognizing the importance of mental well-being demonstrates self-awareness and a commitment to personal growth. It's a positive and empowering choice on the journey towards mental health and overall well-being.

Chapter 8: Integrating Mindfulness into Daily Life

This chapter is dedicated to introducing readers to the transformative power of mindfulness and providing practical ways to incorporate it into their daily routines.

Mindful Living Practices

To integrate mindful living into daily life:

Start Small: Begin with short, focused moments of mindfulness. Gradually expand as it becomes more natural.

Morning Routine: Incorporate mindfulness into your morning routine. Practice mindful breathing, stretching, or gratitude to set a positive tone for the day.

Tech Breaks: Take short breaks from screens. Use these moments for mindful breathing or a brief walk to refresh your mind.

Mindful Breathing: Practice conscious breathing throughout the day. Focus on your breath to bring yourself into the present moment.

Nature Connection: Spend time in nature. Whether a walk in the park or simply observing the outdoors, connect with the environment mindfully.

Mindful Transitions: Be present during transitions between tasks. Take a moment to breathe and reset before moving to the next activity.

Mindful Listening: Practice active listening in conversations. Be fully present and engaged without distractions.

Body Scan: Occasionally check in with your body. Notice areas of tension and consciously release any stress.

Evening Reflection: Reflect on the day before bed. Consider moments of gratitude and acknowledge challenges with self-compassion.

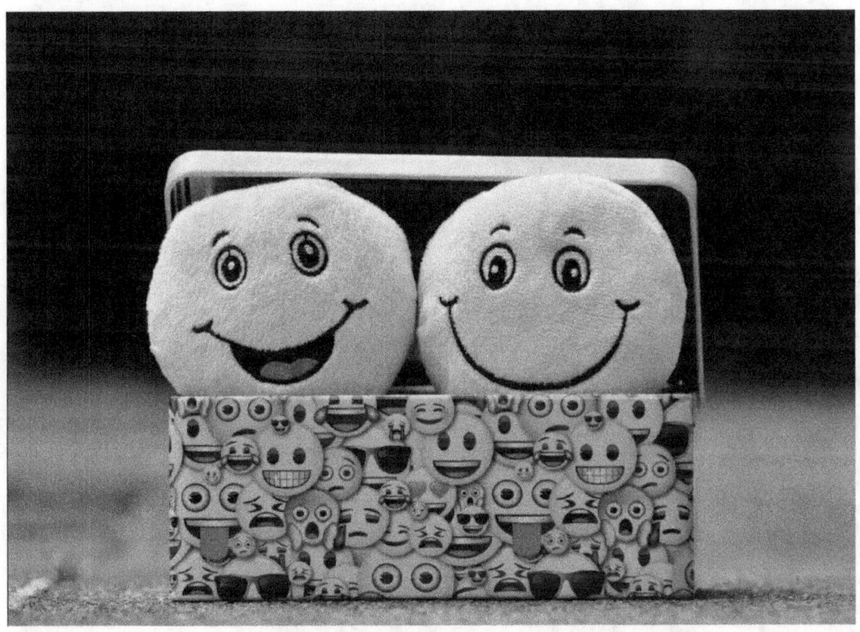

Mindful Eating and Mindful Movement

To integrate mindful eating and mindful movement into daily life:

Mindful Eating:

Savor Each Bite: Eat slowly and savor each bite. Pay attention to flavors, textures, and the overall experience of eating.

Eliminate Distractions: Minimize distractions like TV or phone during meals. Focus solely on the act of eating.

Portion Awareness: Be mindful of portion sizes. Listen to your body's hunger and fullness cues.

Chew Mindfully: Chew your food thoroughly. This not only aids digestion but also allows you to fully experience the taste.

Gratitude Practice: Before eating, take a moment to express gratitude for the food in front of you.

Mindful Snacking: Extend mindfulness to snacks. Choose nourishing options and be present while enjoying them.

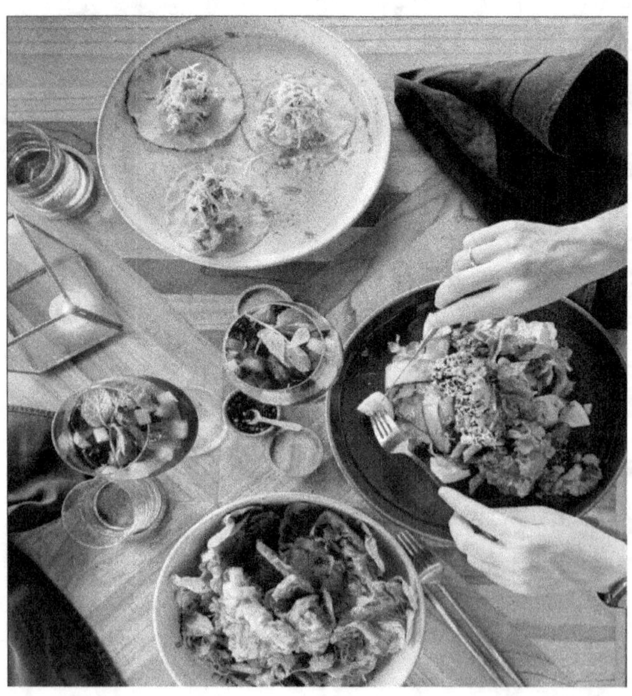

***Mindful Movement:**

Choose Enjoyable Activities: Engage in physical activities you enjoy. It could be walking, yoga, dancing, or any form of exercise that brings you joy.

Focus on Sensations: During movement, pay attention to the sensations in your body. Notice the rhythm of your breath and the feeling of your muscles working

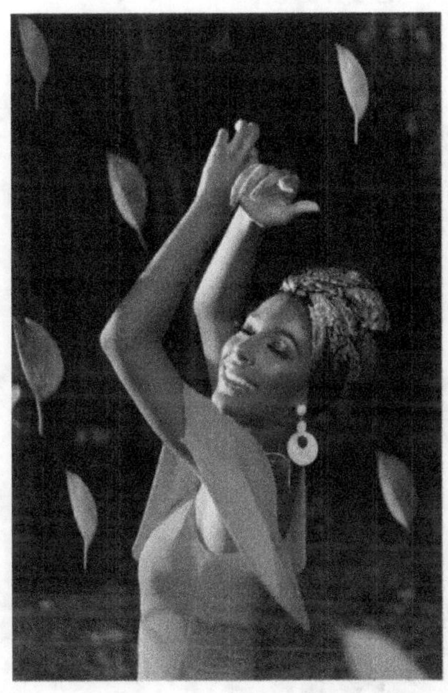
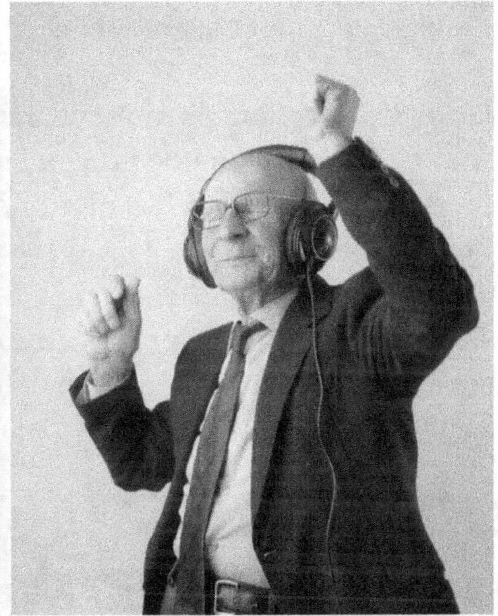

Mindfulness for Stress Reduction:

  To integrate mindfulness for stress reduction into daily life:

Start with Breathing: Practice mindful breathing exercises. Take short breaks to focus on deep, intentional breaths to calm the nervous system.

Morning Mindfulness Routine: Begin the day with a few minutes of mindfulness. This could include meditation, mindful stretching, or setting positive intentions.

Mindful Breaks: Take short breaks throughout the day to engage in mindfulness. This could be a brief walk, a few moments of deep breathing, or a mindful pause before transitioning between tasks.

Body Scan Meditation: Incorporate a body scan meditation into your routine. This involves bringing awareness to each part of your body, releasing tension as you go.

Nature Connection: Spend time in nature mindfully. Whether it's a walk in the park or simply observing the outdoors, connect with the environment and let it be a source of tranquility.

Mindful Listening: Be present in conversations. Practice active listening without immediately formulating responses in your mind.

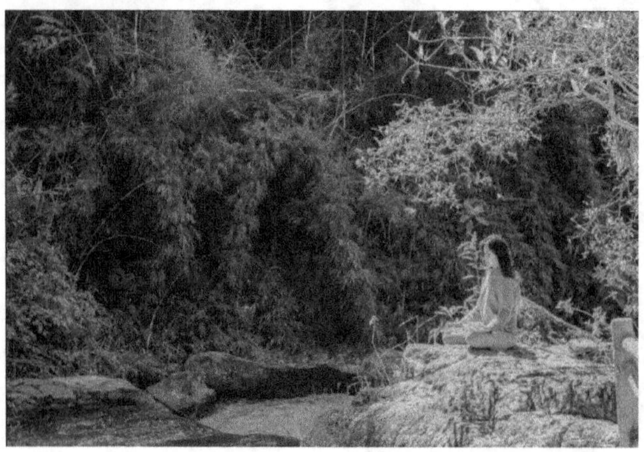

Evening Reflection: Before bed, engage in a brief mindfulness reflection. Acknowledge the positive aspects of your day and let go of any stressors.

Mindful Technology Use: Be mindful of your screen time. Take breaks from electronic devices and use technology intentionally, avoiding mindless scrolling.

Gratitude Practice: Cultivate a gratitude practice. Regularly take a moment to reflect on things you are thankful for, fostering a positive mindset.

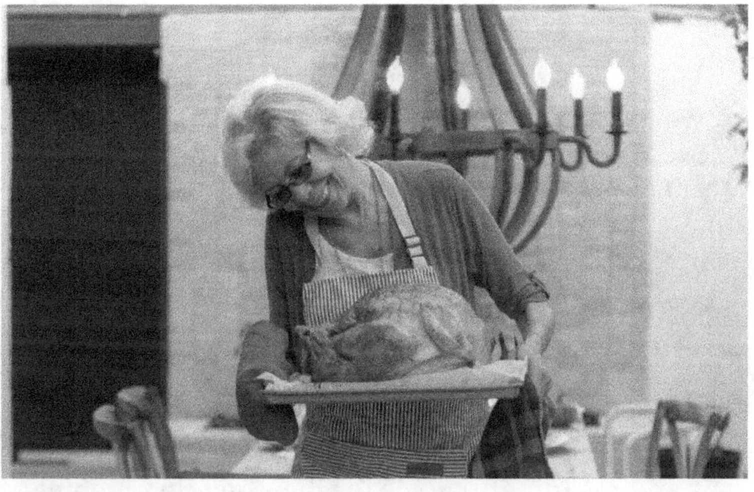

Consistency is key. Integrate these practices gradually, adapting them to your preferences and schedule. Over time, mindfulness can become a natural and effective tool for stress reduction in your daily life

Chapter 9: Embracing Continuous Growth

This chapter focuses on the idea that mental health is an ongoing journey of growth and self-discovery. It covers:

Reflecting on Progress:

- Reflect on your mental health journey and celebrate achievements, no matter how small.
- Appreciate the importance of recognizing and learning from setbacks.

Lifelong Learning and Adaptability:

- Emphasize the ever-evolving nature of mental health strategies, urging yourself to stay open to new approaches and information.
- Explore the concept of lifelong learning and its positive impact on mental well-being.

Setting New Goals:

- Set realistic and meaningful goals for their ongoing mental health journey.
- Know the value of having both short-term and long-term goals.

Connecting with a Community:

- Recognize the importance of building a supportive community or joining mental health groups to share experiences and insights.
- Explore the benefits of mutual support in sustaining

mental well-being.

This chapter serves as a bridge between the practical strategies discussed earlier and the concluding remarks, reinforcing the idea that mental health is a dynamic process that involves continuous learning, adaptation, and personal growth.

Conclusion:

As we reach the culmination of "Mindful Mastery: A Guide to Mental Health Strategies," let's revisit the key strategies that form the foundation of this journey towards enhanced well-being.

1. Recap of Key Strategies:
  - *Mind-Body Connection:* Acknowledge the profound link between mental and physical health, fostering a holistic approach.

  - *Embracing Emotions:* Cultivate a healthy relationship with emotions, recognizing them as integral to the human experience.

  - *Cognitive Strategies:* Equip yourself with cognitive tools like CBT and mindfulness, empowering you to navigate life's challenges.

  - *Social Connections:* Understand the vital role of supportive relationships and effective communication in promoting mental wellness.

  - *Lifestyle Factors:* Prioritize sleep, nutrition, and exercise—cornerstones of a resilient and balanced mental state.

  - *Professional Help:* Recognize the strength in seeking therapy and, when necessary, integrating medication as part of your mental health toolkit.

  - *Mindfulness Practices:* Embrace mindfulness in daily

living, from mindful eating to incorporating mindful movement into your routine.

2. Encouragement for Ongoing Mental Health Maintenance:

   As you embark on the continuous journey of mental health maintenance:
   - *Reflect on Progress:* Celebrate your achievements, big and small, and acknowledge the progress made.

   - *Embrace Lifelong Learning:* Stay open to evolving strategies, recognizing that mental well-being is a lifelong journey of learning and adaptation.

   - *Set New Goals:* Establish realistic and meaningful goals, fostering a sense of purpose and direction.

   - *Connect with Community:* Cultivate connections with a supportive community, sharing experiences and insights that contribute to collective well-being.

   - *Recognize its an ongoing effort:* Knowing that mental health is an ongoing journey of growth and self-discovery is The master strategy that really existed.

In closing, remember that the pursuit of mental health is not a destination but a dynamic process. Your commitment to ongoing maintenance is a testament to your resilience and strength. As you apply these strategies in your daily life, may you find a profound and lasting sense of mindful mastery, creating a foundation for a healthier and more fulfilling existence.